7 Reasons to Straighten Your Teeth

David S. Ostreicher, DDS, MS, MPH

David S. Ostreicher, DDS,MS,MPH
7 Reasons to Straighten Your Teeth

Invisalign® is a registered trademark of Align Technology, Inc.
The information in this book is designed to help you make informed decisions about your dental health. It should be used only in conjunction with guidance and care from your dentist or orthodontist.
7reasons.info

Copyright © 2010 Dr. David S. Ostreicher
All rights reserved.

ISBN: 145156239X
ISBN-13: 9781451562392

Contents

Introduction: Malocclusion Is a Disease 1

Chapter 1: Look Better 3

Chapter 2: Healthier Teeth 21

Chapter 3: Feel Better 39

Chapter 4: Live Longer 55

Chapter 5: Smell Better 67

Chapter 6: It's No Accident 81

Chapter 7: Unexpected Benefits: 97
      (The *Invisalign*® **Advantage**)

This book is dedicated to all the fine folks out there whose quality of life and appearance would be dramatically improved if only they would straighten their teeth.

"Every human being is the author of his own health or disease."

—*Hindu Prince Gautama Siddharta, the founder of Buddhism, 563–483 B.C.*

Introduction

MALOCCLUSION IS A DISEASE.

Disease is defined medically as *"incorrectly functioning organ, part, structure, or system of the body"** or *"atypical variations of structure and function"***

Malocclusion means, literally, *"bad bite."* When your teeth are crowded, or spaced too far apart, or are crooked, or don't mesh together correctly, you have malocclusion. You might not think of malocclusion as a disease, but it is, and malocclusion is a condition that causes other health problems.

Like most diseases, early detection and treatment of malocclusion usually is the most effective approach. And like many diseases, if left untreated, malocclusion generally becomes worse with time. Fortunately, malocclusion can now easily be treated at any age.

Unlike many diseases, malocclusion is usually easy to diagnose, even if you're not a dentist. You probably have a pretty good idea about whether your teeth are crooked or spaced. So does anyone who looks at you. They can tell at a glance if your teeth are crowded or bucked or spaced. But they're probably too polite to say anything to you. That doesn't mean that they don't know that you have malocclusion disease. They are just wondering why you don't have it treated!

*dictionary.com
**Wikipedia

7 REASONS TO STRAIGHTEN YOUR TEETH

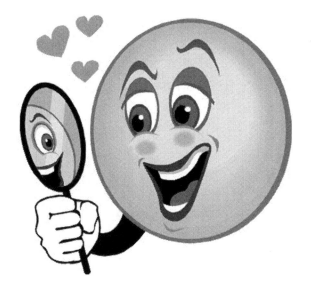

1. Look Better

When you have crowded, crooked teeth, your whole facial appearance is affected. You don't look your best, and your good features are overshadowed by your misaligned teeth. Your smile is the first thing others notice when they look at you. Your ability to make a good first impression at a job interview or on a date might be limited by your crooked teeth—and if you don't make a good first impression, you might not get a second chance. Fortunately, today straightening your teeth as an adult can be done easily, painlessly, and best of all, invisibly. You can look better in a matter of months.

7 REASONS TO STRAIGHTEN YOUR TEETH

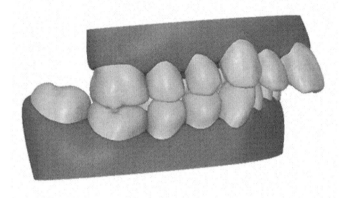

1. LOOK BETTER

BUCK TEETH

If your upper teeth stick way out in front of your lower teeth, then you have buck teeth, or, to use the medical term, you have *overjet*. Cartoons of rabbits and beavers often exaggerate their buck teeth. The cartoons may be cute, but buck teeth aren't so cute in people, especially adults.

Buck teeth can disturb your entire facial profile. When your front teeth jet out, they force your upper lip forward. That can make you look like you have an underdeveloped chin. Buck teeth can also cause premature tooth wear and increase your risk of cavities. They also make it difficult or even painful to bite down on hard foods, such as apples and carrots.

With the upper front teeth trying to escape from the mouth, the lower front teeth have nothing to bite against. This can cause the lower front teeth to *over-erupt* (come too far out of their socket), and bang into the *palate* (roof of the mouth). This is called an *overbite*.

7 REASONS TO STRAIGHTEN YOUR TEETH

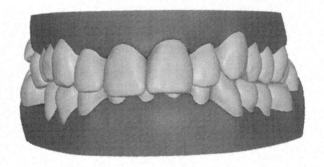

1. LOOK BETTER

OVERBITE

Normally, your upper teeth overlap your lower teeth by only a millimeter or two. If you could look inside your mouth while it's closed, you should see that the biting edge of your top front teeth covers your lower teeth by just a little bit. Anything more than that is an *overbite*.

Often, an overbite is so severe that the lower teeth are actually biting into the palate. When this happens, the lower teeth are not visible when smiling; they are completely obscured by the upper teeth. Not only does this look awkward, but as the lower teeth stab the palate, they can cause inflammation in the gums behind the upper front teeth—and that can lead to gum disease or tooth loss.

A severe overbite can sometimes cause muscle spasms, headaches or pain in the *tempromandibular joint*. (The joint that attaches your lower jaw to your skull)

Sometimes an overbite is referred to as a "deep bite."

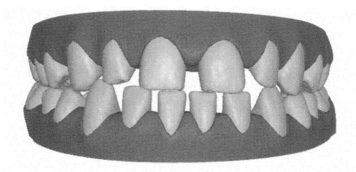

SPACED TEETH

Shark teeth are normally spaced, which is perfect for their all flesh diet. People teeth are normally touching each other, which suits our more varied diet. Unless you eat like a shark, you want your teeth touching each other.

Teeth ordinarily touch each other in an area called the *contact point*. Usually the contact point is a very small area, just 1 or 2 square millimeters. If you're wise enough to use dental floss on a daily basis, the floss should snap through the contact point easily as you apply slight pressure. If teeth aren't touching at the contact point, then you have spaced teeth.

Spaced teeth not only look funny, but food can become stuck in the spaces between them, leading to periodontal disease or cavities. Normal teeth that are touching each other are stabilized, and can better withstand the forces of chewing. Spaced teeth are more likely to become loose from uneven chewing forces.

Spaced teeth can sometimes cause various types of speech pathology.

7 REASONS TO STRAIGHTEN YOUR TEETH

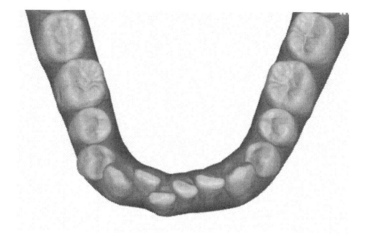

CROWDED TEETH

Crowded teeth are a common dental problem. Sometimes, there's just not enough room along the jawbone for the teeth to be evenly positioned. Sometimes, teeth seem to be too big for the jaws. This can be a genetic malocclusion—you might inherit big teeth from one parent, yet small jaw bones from your other parent.

Often, teeth tend to become more crowded as you get older. As teeth become more crowded, they become increasingly more twisted and turned. Orthodontists call this adult onset mandibular crowding when it occurs in the lower jaw. This can become so severe that the crowding forces one or more teeth out of the normal arch of the jaw. Adult onset mandibular crowding is very common—about 65 percent of all adult Americans have it.

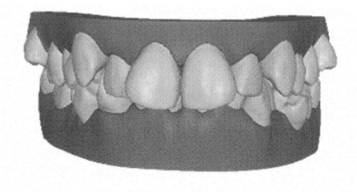

CROOKED TEETH

If you constantly have a tight-lipped smile, it's probably because you're trying not to show your crooked teeth.

Crooked teeth are a combination of crowding and twisting. Not only do they look bad, but crooked teeth are very difficult to care for.

Crooked teeth have overlapping contact points that have a larger than usual area. That makes it harder to keep the teeth clean by brushing and flossing.

Crooked teeth can make you look old and mean. And who wants to look old and mean?

7 REASONS TO STRAIGHTEN YOUR TEETH

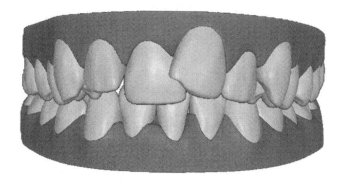

SLANTED TEETH

Do your teeth slant to the right or to the left? Is your upper midline centered with the midline of your face? If not, then you have slanted teeth.

Slanted teeth look unsymmetrical and lopsided. Often, missing teeth causes slanted teeth. If a tooth is missing, the other teeth tend to slant toward the missing space in an attempt to close the gap. Nature abhors a vacuum.

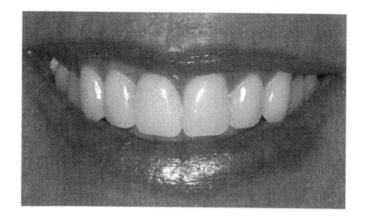

STRAIGHT TEETH LOOK WHITER

Crooked, crowded and slanted teeth tend to look dull and dim. They reflect light differently, and often look dark or shady.

Even if you have your teeth professionally bleached or whitened, they will look gray and dark if they are crooked or crowded.

Straight teeth reflect light more evenly and cast no shadows. Straight teeth look white and bright.

The bacteria that cause tooth decay can also cause swollen, bleeding gums.

NICER GUMS

When you look in the mirror, do you want to see nice, straight white teeth, or crooked teeth and puffy red gums?

Crowded teeth, crooked teeth, overjet and overbite can all lead to swollen, red, bleeding gums because it is very difficult to keep maloccluded teeth and the gums around them clean. Often the gums can appear so large and swollen that they actually obscure your teeth. When you straighten your teeth, your gums are very likely to improve as well.

Some malocclusions, such as an overbite, may cause a "gummy smile". When you smile or talk, you flash a wall of gums instead of your pearly whites. Orthodontic treatment can often correct this.

2. Healthier Teeth

Healthy teeth look good and feel good—and straight teeth are healthier, look better, and feel better than crooked or crowded teeth. Straight teeth get fewer cavities and are less likely to have problems such as discoloration, uneven wear and fractures. The gums around straight teeth are also healthier and less likely to develop periodontal disease. When your teeth are healthy, your smile is much nicer. The teeth appear whiter, they have fewer fillings, and the gums that hold them in place are pink and even. What about feeling good? Straight teeth and healthy gums mean you can easily chew anything you want. Your teeth are less likely to be sensitive to heat or cold and you're at much lower risk of developing painful dental problems.

7 REASONS TO STRAIGHTEN YOUR TEETH

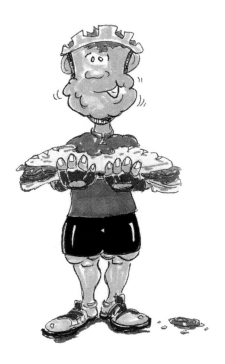

STRAIGHT TEETH CHEW BETTER

Did you know that your body has no enzymes that can break down the cell walls of carrots, peppers, tomatoes, apples or any other plants? That is because all plant cells have tough, cellulose cell walls that cannot be digested by your normal digestive juices. To fully digest raw fruits and vegetables you must bite through the cell walls with your teeth. And if your bite is off, your chewing ability may be inadequate.

Scientists who study chewing ability call this "masticatory proficiency." People who have maloccluded teeth with poor masticatory proficiency are more likely to develop some forms of malnutrition and digestive disturbances.

So, if you like to munch on fresh fruits and vegetables, it is important to have a good bite!

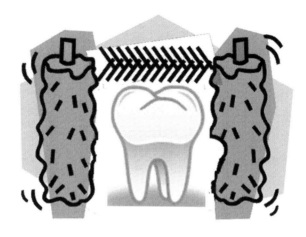

The average human produces 25,000 quarts of saliva in a lifetime. That is enough saliva to fill two swimming pools!

STRAIGHT TEETH ARE SELF CLEANING

Think of your mouth as an automatic car wash. Well, actually a tooth wash.

You've got three pairs of major salivary glands (parotid, sublingual, and submandibular) in your mouth, along with hundreds of minor salivary glands. They're like the water spray in the car wash—they continuously bathe your teeth in saliva. While there's no soap in saliva, it still does a great job of keeping your teeth clean. Your saliva is neutral—not too acid or alkaline. It's loaded with antibodies, enzymes and other agents that are designed to kill the germs that cause cavities and bad breath. You might think of your saliva as just spit, but your teeth think of it as their natural environment.

Straight teeth have all of their surfaces exposed to the constant washing action of saliva. Crooked teeth don't. Saliva can't get into the tight spaces between crowded, overlapping teeth very well, which means it can't wash out the bacteria and food debris that gets stuck in there.

Your lips and tongue are the brushes of your tooth wash machinery. As you talk and swallow, your lips polish the outside surfaces of your teeth and your tongue polishes the inside surfaces. But if your teeth are crowded or crooked, your natural brushes will miss large surface areas of your teeth. These areas will collect food debris and bacteria. All that soft, gelatinous, gooey material becomes *plaque*, a thin film that sticks to our teeth and causes cavities, periodontal disease and bad breath.

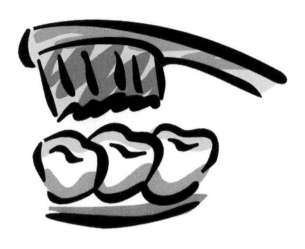

Boar, badger and horse hair were used for toothbrush bristles but were later found to be abrasive and harsh.

The first nylon bristled toothbrush with a plastic handle was invented in 1938.

STRAIGHT TEETH ARE EASIER TO BRUSH

Toothbrush manufacturers would have a much easier time if everyone had straight teeth. Toothbrush bristles have no difficulty in navigating large, broad open spaces. But toothbrush bristles have a great challenge when cleaning in between crowded, overlapping crooked teeth. In order to navigate in between these teeth, the bristles have to be made thinner and more flexible. But the thinner and more flexible the bristles, the less effective they are at removing plaque.

Toothbrush manufacturers call this *interproximal access efficacy*. (Interproximal is the official scientific term for in between teeth). If the teeth are overlapping, it is nearly impossible for toothbrush bristles to clean the area thoroughly, no matter what kind of bristles the brush has.

If your teeth are straight, then it will be much easier to keep them clean using a toothbrush. The bristles will more easily find their way into the nooks and crannies in between your teeth. Your teeth will be cleaner, you will suffer fewer cavities, have less periodontal disease, and your breath will be fresher.

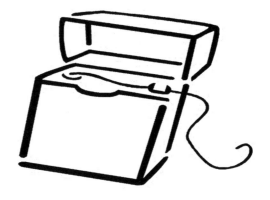

Over three million miles of dental floss is purchased in North America each year!

STRAIGHT TEETH ARE EASIER TO FLOSS

Dental floss is the most effective way to clean in between your teeth.

People use dental floss for all sorts of other things as well—it's very versatile. You can use it as a thread to sew a button, to hang pictures, and as fishing line. You can even make emergency toilet repairs with it. But because it can be so frustrating to use in your mouth, people often give up on using dental floss for its primary purpose.

Flossing straight teeth requires a great deal of manual dexterity. The floss should maneuver in between the contact points of adjacent teeth. It should then be wrapped around the side of one tooth and moved up and down in a cleaning motion, to be repeated on the adjacent tooth. But when teeth are crooked or crowded, flossing gets much more difficult. The floss snags, shreds and tears, making the entire procedure as difficult as removing the clamshell packaging on the four-pack of toothpaste you purchased at *Costco*.

Even with nice, straight teeth, nearly 35 percent of a tooth's surface is not readily accessible by toothbrush bristles. That number grows significantly if teeth are crowded or crooked. That makes dental floss even more important.

7 REASONS TO STRAIGHTEN YOUR TEETH

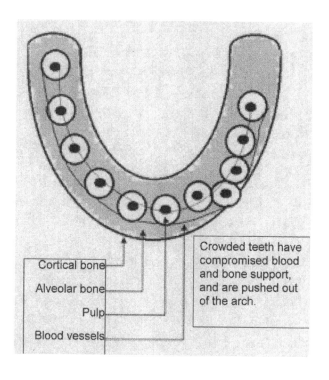

2. HEALTHIER TEETH

ON THE BONE

Your teeth are held to your jawbones in a very complicated fashion. Both your upper jaw (maxilla) and lower jaw (mandible) have troughs that your teeth are attached to. The center of the trough is soft, spongy *alveolar* bone. This bone has a rich blood and nerve supply that feeds the blood supply of your tooth (*pulp*).

Surrounding the alveolar bone, on the front and back surfaces of your teeth, is the thick, *cortical* bone. Cortical bone, while thicker and stronger than alveolar bone has a very limited blood supply.

Straight teeth are normally situated in the center of the alveolar bone trough, where they are happily bathed in a rich blood supply of oxygen and nutrients.

Crowded teeth can push teeth out of the alveolar trough, into the cortical bone. This can compromise the blood supply to the tooth and its surrounding tissues. Even scarier, when teeth are really crowded, they can be pushed out of the alveolar trough, through the cortical bone and through the gums. This causes the root of the tooth to be exposed. It makes you look "long in the tooth" which is unattractive. The real problem, though, is that teeth with exposed roots are very vulnerable to decay and damage, meaning you could lose the tooth.

7 REASONS TO STRAIGHTEN YOUR TEETH

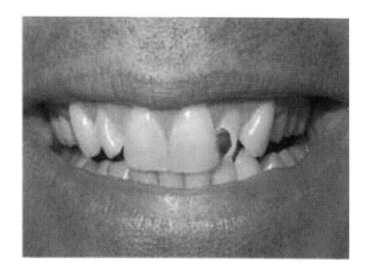

Mick Jagger of The Rolling Stones had an emerald chip placed in his upper right central incisor. But he switched to a diamond when everyone mistook the costly green stone for a piece of spinach.

FOOD IMPACTION

Alligators eat nothing but meat—along with skin, fur and bones—but rarely get any of it impacted (stuck) in between their teeth. That is fortunate for the alligator, because when meat or other foods get stuck in between the teeth, it makes the perfect setup for bacteria. They love it in there. It's nice and warm, it's wet and dark, and there's plenty of food. The bacteria move right in and start eating the impacted food, or, in other words, the impacted food between your teeth begins to rot. That gives the alligator—or you—bad breath and cavities, to say nothing of inflamed gums and periodontal disease.

Fortunately for alligators, their teeth are pointy, and positioned at a distance from each other, so alligators don't get food impaction. But you're no alligator—your back teeth are wide and broad. Normally, they're lined up next to each other, touching at only a small *contact point*. This elegant design limits food impaction. But if your teeth are crooked or crowded, the areas between the teeth are far more susceptible to retaining food debris—and it's much harder to brush and floss the debris away.

Food impaction can cause swelling of the gums, and be a very painful condition. Plus, a piece of impacted steak or tuna fish can really turn a beautiful smile into a yucky disgusting mess!

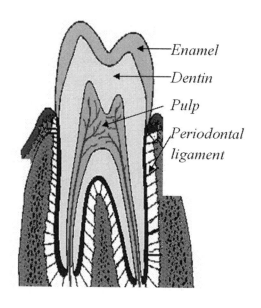

2. HEALTHIER TEETH

BETTER BLOOD FLOW

Your teeth are living, breathing things. Well, they don't actually breathe, but they do require oxygen which they get from the rich blood supply of the surrounding jaw bone.

Your teeth are attached to your jawbone by the *periodontal ligament*. This is a hammock of elastic fibers that suspend your teeth in their sockets. Unlike most ligaments in your body, the periodontal ligament has capillaries and a rather substantial blood flow.

The blood flow in the periodontal ligament is connected to the blood flow in your tooth. In the center of your tooth is the *pulp*, which is made up of nerves and blood vessels. Surrounding your pulp is a type of living tissue called *dentin*, and surrounding that is the *enamel*— the very tough, white outer layer of the tooth. Enamel is inorganic—it doesn't have a blood supply and if it's damaged, say by a cavity, it doesn't grow back.

The pulp services your teeth, bringing oxygen and nutrients to the dentin. The pulp also has nerves, which allow you to feel the cold of ice cream and the warmth of hot cocoa.

Crooked or crowded teeth fight for the available space within your jawbone. The roots of the teeth can press on each other's periodontal ligament and choke the blood supply. On some occasions, the battle is so severe, that one or both of the pressing roots can be severely damaged. This can cause *root resorption*, where your own body attacks and destroys the roots—and that could eventually lead to the loss of one or more teeth.

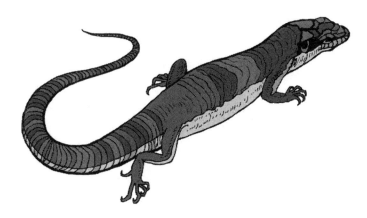

The Komodo dragon's mouth is full of virulent bacteria and even if its prey survives the original bite, it will die of infection later from the dragon's poisonous tooth bacteria.

LESS TOXIC BACTERIA

You were born with a sterile mouth. But when your mom gave you your first kiss, she inoculated you with bacteria! Since then your mouth has been populated with billions and billions of bacteria. That's perfectly normal. Most of the bacteria are harmless, but some cause cavities, periodontal disease, bad breath, and perhaps even some types of oral cancers.

Your mouth is the perfect breeding place for bacteria. It is warm and moist and has a constant source of nutrients, including doughnuts, sugary drinks and pasta, to name a few. Good brushing and flossing will help to remove some of the bacteria from your teeth and gums, but you will always leave a few million behind.

Germs come in two varieties: *aerobic* (bacteria that need oxygen) and *anaerobic* (bacteria that thrive in the absence of oxygen). The aerobic kind in general seem to be relatively harmless, but the anaerobic variety are far more virulent and destructive. The excretions of anaerobic bacteria destroy the periodontal ligament and cause inflammation of the gums.

Crowded teeth are a perfect environment for the harmful anaerobic bacteria. The hampered blood supply to crowded teeth, and the irregular gum tissues surrounding them, reduces the oxygen in the area and encourages bacterial growth. Straightening your teeth improves the blood flow and increases the oxygen level, which makes it harder for anaerobic bacteria to colonize your mouth.

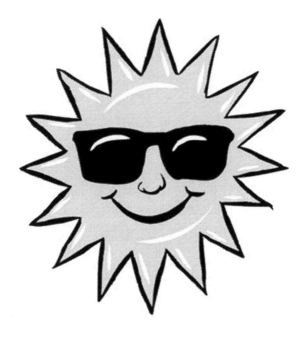

3. Feel Better

In addition to all the physical benefits of straightening your teeth, there's another reason that is perhaps even more important: You'll feel better about yourself.

Let's face it, appearances matter. Much as we know we should judge people by their character, not their appearance, unconsciously we often do make negative judgments based only on how someone looks. And if your teeth aren't in good shape, you yourself could be the victim of a negative snap judgment. That appearance-based decision, even when it's unconscious, could mean that you don't get that second job interview, or that you don't make that big sale, or that you don't get asked out for another date. It's possible that your misaligned teeth are holding you back in both your professional and personal life.

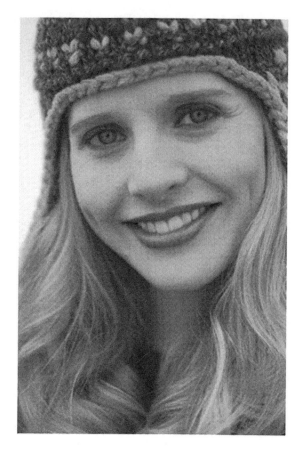

"A smile is something you can't give away; it always comes back to you."

NICE SMILES MAKE A DIFFERENCE

A major study in 2007 involving more than five hundred people compared pictures of people before and after they had their teeth straightened. Half the participants were shown a set of pictures of smiling people. Some of them had fixed their teeth and some hadn't; the participants didn't know which were which. The other participants were shown exactly the same set of pictures, but the before and after shots were reversed. The participants were asked to rate the people in the pictures based only on their appearance. Across the board, they rated the people with nice smiles—defined by straight white teeth—as more attractive, intelligent, happy, successful in their career, friendly, interesting, kind, wealthy, and popular with the opposite sex. The people in the both sets of pictures were the same—the only difference was in their smiles. The study shows that a nice smile has a big impact on how others perceive your personality and your attractiveness.

7 REASONS TO STRAIGHTEN YOUR TEETH

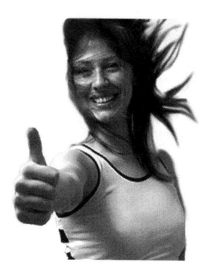

SELF-ESTEEM AND SELF-CONFIDENCE

The judgments of others aren't the only problem. Knowing that your teeth are crowded or crooked can also have a severe impact on your self esteem. You might be very self-conscious about smiling, laughing, or even speaking, because these actions will reveal your dental problems. Having a constant source of concern and embarrassment in your life lowers your self-esteem. How can you feel good about yourself when one of the most visible parts of you is an embarrassment? How can you have the self-confidence to speak up for yourself if you're ashamed to show your teeth? How can you have any real fun if you don't want to smile or laugh in public?

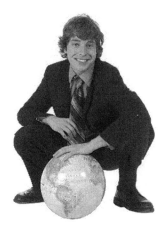

ADULT SELF-ESTEEM

The self-esteem issues you might have from your dental appearance may date back many years. As a typical teenager you probably agonized over your dental appearance; you might also have been teased about your teeth. Not so great for building your self-esteem and confidence during those crucial adolescent years. As an adult, you may still feel bad about your teeth. Maybe people don't tease you about your teeth anymore, but the memory of that teasing and that teenage agony is still with you. Because your teeth are still such an important part of your appearance and how people perceive you, you feel bad about yourself.

7 REASONS TO STRAIGHTEN YOUR TEETH

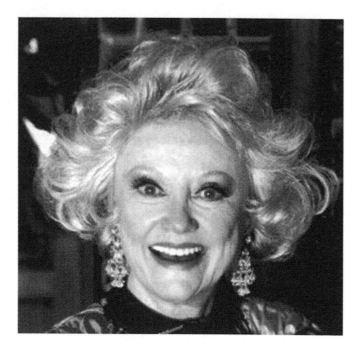

"A smile is a curve that sets everything straight."
Phyllis Diller

SELF-ESTEEM AND SELF-DEFEATING BEHAVIOR

Low self-esteem from misaligned teeth can lead to a downward spiral of self-defeating behavior. Because you're embarrassed about your teeth, you do things, like smiling with your mouth closed and not laughing much, that may make people think you're cold and unfriendly. They may react negatively, which only lowers your self esteem. Feeling self-conscious about your teeth leads you to self-defeating actions that cover up your true abilities. You might be embarrassed about public speaking, for instance, thinking that all eyes will be on your crooked teeth. Your reluctance to speak in public, however, means that you might not get the recognition you deserve. It could also mean that you don't get a promotion to a job that requires making a lot of presentations. Nothing crashes your self-esteem like being ignored or getting turned down for a promotion.

Correcting those crooked teeth means never having to hide your smile again. You can truly be yourself at last. You'll gain the self-confidence and self-esteem that are crucial for success.

positive
negative

TURNING NEGATIVES INTO POSITIVES

People with crooked or missing teeth are often perceived negatively. They're judged by stereotypes that say bad teeth mean you're poor and ignorant, or too lazy to bother brushing your teeth, or that you don't care about your appearance. Because we judge so much by appearances, people with missing teeth may find that they face major barriers to personal and professional success.

The same is true of teeth that are badly maloccluded. Unfair as these judgments might be, they're also a fact of life. People with crowded and crooked teeth are often perceived as being poor or uneducated—even not that smart. This sort of bias against you can really hold you back in social and business settings.

Straightening your teeth, and also resolving any other dental issues, such as missing teeth, can do a lot to change the way you're seen by people who meet you for the first time. You'll make a much better first impression. The negative perception will be replaced by a positive one. Instead of focusing on your maloccluded teeth, people will focus on you as a person.

7 REASONS TO STRAIGHTEN YOUR TEETH

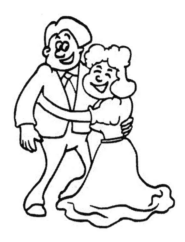

ATTRACTIVE SMILES ARE ATTRACTIVE

A really influential study about dental appearance in children appeared in the *American Journal of Orthodontics* back in 1981. In this study, the same photos of two boys and two girls were modified (this was long before *Photoshop*) so that there were five different versions for each face. In each version, the child's face was the same but the teeth were changed. The appearance of the children ran from normal, all the way up to severely crowded teeth. The pictures were shown randomly to over eighty people, who were asked to rate how attractive each child was. Just about everyone who saw the face with the nicest teeth rated the child as being friendly, attractive, smart, and desirable as a friend. You've probably already guessed that the child with the most severely maloccluded teeth was seen as less attractive, more aggressive, not as smart, and not very desirable as a friend.

This study was of kids, but adults know that appearance is a big part of social attractiveness at all ages. That isn't to say only beautiful people can have a good social life. What it does say, however, is that off-putting physical characteristics, such as crowded and crooked teeth, can give the wrong impression about you and limit your social life even as a grown-up.

7 REASONS TO STRAIGHTEN YOUR TEETH

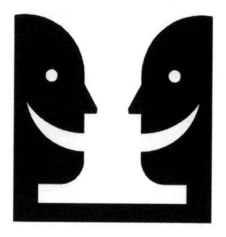

HAPPY SMILES ARE CONTAGIOUS

Even if you smile a lot, how you smile makes a difference in how you're perceived. We know from many psychological studies of expressions and body language that a closed, tight-lipped smile—the sort of smile you might have if you're self-conscious about your misaligned teeth—is often perceived incorrectly by others. You might well be happy, but to them, your closed smile means you're not. An upper smile—meaning you're showing only your upper teeth—is seen as friendlier and more happy. If your bottom teeth are the problem, you might be willing to show an upper smile. If your top teeth are the problem, though, there's no such thing as a bottom smile—you're stuck with the unfriendly-seeming closed smile. Of course, the studies also show that a true broad smile showing your top and bottom teeth is seen as the friendliest, happiest, and most attractive smile of all. Does this work the other way? If you straighten your teeth so you can smile broadly without being self-conscious, will this make you happier and more attractive? Well, other people will think you are, and that will give your self-esteem a big boost. And smiling is contagious—the more you flash your new broad smile, the more people will smile back at you, and that will make you smile even more.

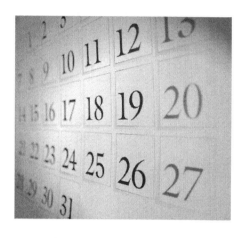

4. Live Longer

We know that straightening your teeth can reduce your risk of serious dental problems, and we know it can make you look better and feel better about yourself. What we've also learned in recent years is that fixing your teeth could actually help you live a longer, healthier life.

Does this sound too good to be true? It's not. Let's look at the many ways that straighter teeth and improved dental health can lead to improved overall health.

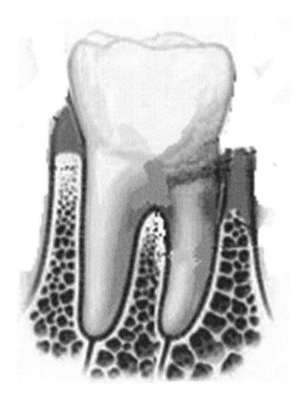

The right side of this tooth has periodontal disease. The gums are inflamed, and the level of bone has deteriorated.

REDUCE PERIODONTAL DISEASE

When your teeth are crooked and crowded, it's hard to keep them clean even when you're very diligent about brushing and flossing. Chances are that over time you'll develop periodontal disease. This means that your gums, which hold your teeth in place, get infected. In the most mild form, you develop *gingivitis*: Your gums become red and swollen and bleed easily when you brush your teeth. If gingivitis isn't treated, after a while it can progress to *periodontitis*, which literally means "inflammation around the tooth." The gums pull away from the teeth and form little pockets of infection from trapped food and bacteria. Infection activates your body's immune system, which in turn attacks the bacteria. There's a war going on in your mouth—and all wars cause a lot of damage. The ongoing battle between the bacteria and your immune system can start to break down the gums, connective tissue and bone that hold your teeth in place in your jaw. That can make chewing painful and difficult, and it can lead to teeth that become so loose that they fall out or need to be extracted.

About 80 percent of all Americans have some form of periodontal disease. If you have crooked teeth you're much more likely to not only have gum disease but to have it more seriously.

Gum disease isn't just a problem for your oral health, though. When your mouth is full of harmful bacteria fighting it out with your immune system, your whole body is affected, just as it would be if you had a bad infection on your hand. In particular, the inflammation caused by periodontal disease doesn't affect just your mouth—it can have a very damaging impact on your overall health.

4. LIVE LONGER

DECREASE THE RISK OF HEART DISEASE AND STROKE

Cardiologists (heart doctors) have known for decades that their patients also tend to have dental problems, especially gum disease. An editor's consensus report in a 2009 study published in *The American Journal of Cardiology* showed that people with periodontal disease are 24 percent to 35 percent more likely to suffer coronary artery disease.

What's the connection? There's been a lot of research in this area, and it all seems to come down to inflammation. While inflammation is your body's normal reaction to fight off infection, when inflammation in your mouth goes on for a long time, it can lead to inflammation throughout your body—and that's a well-known risk factor for heart disease. In particular, inflammation is associated with atherosclerosis, or arteries that are narrowed and stiff because they have layers of fatty plaque inside them. When a piece of plaque breaks off or if a blood clot forms, it can block the artery and cause a heart attack; if the plaque or clot gets carried into the blood vessels of the brain, it can cause a stroke. Among older adults, those with gum disease severe enough to cause tooth loss are much more likely to have a stroke than people the same age with healthy gums.

Preventing the inflammation to begin with is the best way to reduce your risk of heart disease and stroke. That means good dental hygiene, but there's a problem. If you have some of the malocclusion problems explained in this book, your risk of gum disease is higher than usual, because you just can't keep your teeth and gums as clean as they need to be to prevent disease. They're too crooked, crowded, or out of position to be brushed and flossed effectively. Straightening your teeth to avoid or help treat gum disease could also help you avoid heart disease. This will help even if you already have gingivitis or periodontitis. In 2007, a research paper in the prestigious *New England Journal of Medicine* showed that intensive periodontal treatment may actually reverse atherosclerosis by making the blood vessels more elastic. Do you feel more like straightening your teeth and keeping them clean after reading this?

DECREASED CANCER RISK

It might sound farfetched to say that there's a connection between tooth brushing and cancer risk, but there definitely is. Periodontal disease seems to be linked to an increased risk of cancer overall, but it's also linked to several types of particularly serious and hard-to-treat cancers, including lung cancer, kidney cancer, and pancreatic cancer. We know this from the famed Health Professionals Follow-Up Study, which has been going on since 1986 and tracks the health of 51,529 American male health professionals aged 40 to 75. In the most recent round of the study, researchers found significant associations between a history of periodontal disease and several cancers, including a 36 percent increase in the risk of lung cancer, a 49 percent increase in the risk of kidney cancer, and a 54 percent increase in the risk of pancreatic cancer. Periodontal disease was also associated with an increased risk of colon cancer, skin melanoma, and some types of blood cancer.

We don't have similar results for women, but the point is obvious: Gum disease is linked to an increased risk of cancer. We can't say yet that solving your gum problems will prevent cancer, but straight teeth and good oral hygiene to prevent and treat periodontal disease is clearly a smart idea.

Low birth weight infants is a leading cause of infant mortality, and costs over $70 billion each year.

PREVENT LOW BIRTH WEIGHT BABIES

More than half a million babies in the United States—about one in eight—are born prematurely, meaning the birth occurs before 37 weeks of pregnancy. Premature babies weigh far less than full-term babies and often require lengthy hospitalization to survive. And even full-term babies can sometimes have low birth weight that causes long-term problems.

In about half of all premature births and low birth weight babies, doctors don't know the cause. One possible reason is periodontal disease in the mother. The reasoning is that the toxins given off by the bacteria have a bad effect on the baby and can trigger premature birth. According to one study, pregnant women who have periodontal disease may be seven times more likely to have a baby that is born too early or too small. There's been a lot of research in this area, and the evidence shows pretty clearly that periodontal disease and pregnancy aren't a good combination. If you're planning to get pregnant, visit your dentist to be checked (and treated if necessary) for periodontal disease. Even if you're already pregnant, treating gum disease is safe and may help prevent a premature or low birth weight baby.

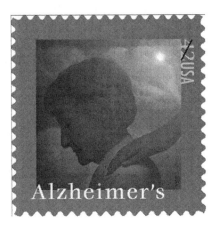

DECREASED RISK OF ALZHEIMER'S DISEASE

Alzheimer's disease, with its relentless loss of mental function, is often seen as an unavoidable risk of growing older. Until recently, there was little evidence that anything could be done to prevent this tragic disease, one that afflicts over five million Americans. Recent research, however, strongly suggests that long-term inflammation starting at a relatively young age can sharply increase the risk of developing Alzheimer's later in life. And that strongly suggests that reducing long-term inflammation could help reduce the risk.

The most exciting study comes from Sweden, where researchers found that exposure to inflammation early in life quadruples the risk of developing Alzheimer's disease. What was one major source of that ongoing inflammation? Periodontal disease. We can't say absolutely that good oral health can prevent Alzheimer's, but we can say that constant inflammation early in life, such as that caused by crooked teeth or chronic gum disease, may have severe consequences later on.

7 REASONS TO STRAIGHTEN YOUR TEETH

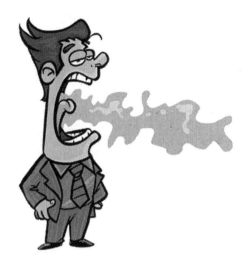

5. Smell Better

Everyone has bad breath now and then, but many people find that they have a continual, serious and embarrassing problem. Studies show that 90 percent of the population has periodic bad breath and 40 percent suffer from chronic bad breath. Unfortunately, oral malodor, commonly known as *halitosis* or bad breath, is socially unacceptable in our hygiene-conscious culture.

7 REASONS TO STRAIGHTEN YOUR TEETH

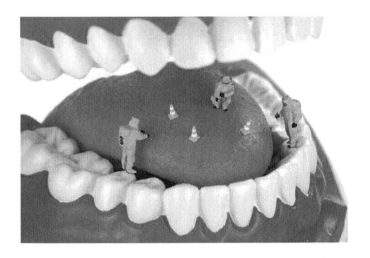

WHAT CAUSES HALITOSIS

More than just a social problem, halitosis is a dental and medical problem. Studies show that 80 percent of halitosis problems originate in the mouth. The remaining 20 percent result from medical causes, such as sinus problems. In the mouth, two factors contribute to bad breath. The areas around the teeth, which are irregular in contour, allow debris to be trapped. Bacteria in the mouth then attack the debris and release bad-smelling gas as they digest it. Similarly, your tongue has a rough surface that entraps gas-producing bacteria.

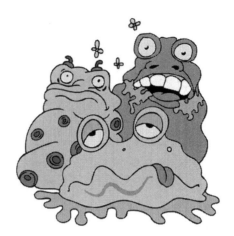

IT'S THE ROTTING FOOD

Whenever you eat, tiny—sometimes microscopic—particles of food get trapped in between your teeth. After several hours, the bacteria that reside in your mouth begin to feast on those leftovers. As the bacteria munch away, the food rots, or putrefies.

Bacteria, like any living organism, give off excretion products as they consume food. Many of these products are foul-smelling gases. With millions and millions of bacteria excreting noxious gases, it's no wonder your breath may not smell sweet.

Crowded or crooked teeth can trap ten times as much food debris as straight teeth. You do the math!

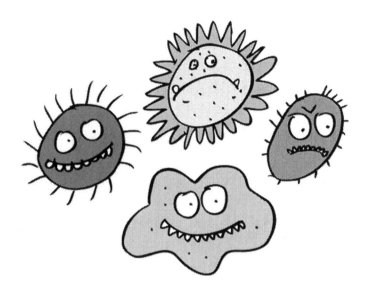

GOOD BACTERIA, BAD BACTERIA

Your mouth contains two classes of bacteria: anaerobic and aerobic. Anaerobic bacteria live in the absence of oxygen. Aerobic bacteria, like you and I, need oxygen. We tend to think of anaerobic bacteria as bad bacteria because their excretions are more toxic than the excretions of aerobic bacteria.

The excretions of anaerobic bacteria are far more destructive to your gum tissues and are the primary cause of periodontal disease. Their secretions are also very high in volatile sulfur compounds—in other words, gases that smell foul, like rotten eggs or sewer gas.

Teeth that are crowded support more anaerobic bacteria growth. Teeth that are straight support more aerobic bacteria growth.

Which bacteria do you want living in your mouth?

7 REASONS TO STRAIGHTEN YOUR TEETH

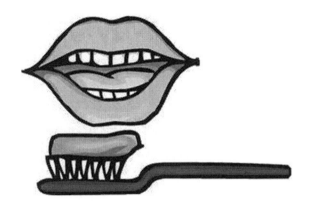

DON'T FORGET YOUR TONGUE

Anaerobic bacteria like to hide out in the nooks and crannies of crowded teeth.

Your tongue also has hills and valleys in the form of *papillae* (taste buds) and taste pores. The same anaerobic bacteria take refuge in the nooks and crannies of your tongue. Even normal tongues in healthy, clean mouths with straight teeth harbor billions of anaerobic bacteria.

So if you want clean breath, brush your teeth often and don't forget to clean your tongue. The most important area to clean is the back center of your tongue, in the center. A toothbrush can't remove tongue bacteria very well. Instead, use a tongue scraper. The best way to do this is with an inexpensive tongue scraper, available at any drugstore. As an alternative, simply use a plastic teaspoon. Place the scraper or spoon on the posterior (back) portion of your tongue and then draw it forward. Be thorough but also gentle. Don't scrape so hard or vigorously that you irritate your tongue.

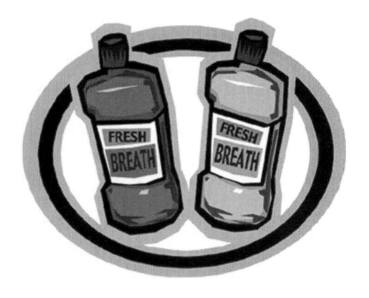

USE A MOUTHWASH

An antibacterial mouth wash can help to kill anaerobic bacteria—but it must be used properly.

The bacteria that are on your teeth, gums and tongue are embedded in a complex biofilm that attach them to each other and to the surfaces in your mouth. In other words, the bacteria are embedded within a self-produced gooey slime, sometimes called plaque. Mouthwash alone can't penetrate the biofilm; you must first break it up with proper tooth brushing, flossing and tongue cleaning. Follow that with your mouthwash, using it according to the manufacturer's directions. That almost always means vigorously swishing the rinse around in your mouth for 30 to 60 seconds. Anything less than that will be ineffective.

7 REASONS TO STRAIGHTEN YOUR TEETH

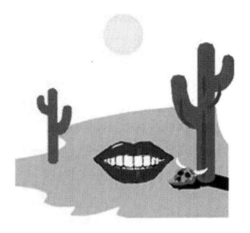

DRY MOUTH

Xerostomia (dry mouth) can lead to an overgrowth of anaerobic bacteria. Saliva naturally contains oxygen and enzymes, which keeps your mouth healthy and fresh, and also washes away bacteria and the food bits they feed on. If you have less saliva, you create an anaerobic environment that's perfect for the bacteria that produce odorous and sour/bitter compounds.

While there are many causes of dry mouth, buck teeth or an open bite can often contribute to this uncomfortable situation. Both of these conditions can lead to mouth breathing while sleeping. Mouth breathing will quickly dry up saliva, causing xerostomia.

7 REASONS TO STRAIGHTEN YOUR TEETH

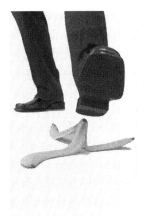

6. It's No Accident

Dentists see the damage accidents can do to teeth all the time. That might not be a top reason for the average person to decide to straighten his or her teeth, but it's one of the main reasons from the dentist's point of view. We've done enough emergency treatments to be very aware of how easily crooked, crowded, or badly spaced teeth can be damaged. Straightening your teeth can help avoid serious accidental injuries to your teeth. A fall off a bike that would be just a bruised lip in someone with straight teeth can be an expensive dental repair for someone with buck teeth, for example. Spend the money to avoid dental accidents rather than treat them.

7 REASONS TO STRAIGHTEN YOUR TEETH

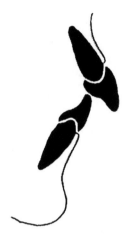

PROTRUDING TEETH

Normally, your upper front teeth should be just one to three millimeters (only an eighth of an inch) in front of your lower front teeth when your mouth is closed. This space is called overjet. If your upper front teeth stick out too far, it is called buck teeth.

Lots of famous "people" have buck teeth—most famously, the cartoon characters Goofy and Sponge Bob Square Pants. These characters illustrate the qualities others often associate with buck teeth: jovial silliness.

If your upper front teeth are sticking out too far, it not only looks funny and gives people the wrong impression of you, it jeopardizes the health and longevity of your teeth. When you have buck teeth protruding from your face, those teeth are dramatically more susceptible to trauma. In fact, an overjet of just five millimeters (only about a quarter of an inch) increases the chances of fracturing your teeth due to trauma by 250 percent!

An overjet of eight millimeters (less than half an inch) raises the risk of fracture due to trauma by a whopping 1,200 percent!

If you like your teeth, tuck them in!

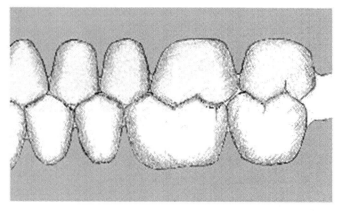

With a good bite, forces are distributed evenly.

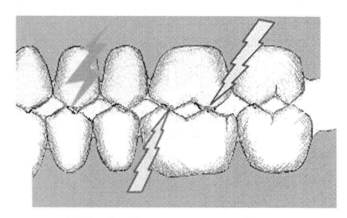

With a bad bite, concentrated forces can cause teeth to fracture.

CLASS II

Which animal can bite with a force of 3,500 pounds per square inch?

a. lion
b. alligator
c. human

Answer: A lion bites with about 700 pounds per square inch. A full-grown, 12-foot alligator can exert about 2,100 pounds when it bites—enough to lift a small pickup truck. The answer is c, humans. Every time you bite down hard on something, you apply 3,500 pounds per square inch of pure force. You put a lot of stress on your teeth every time you chew.

When your occlusion (bite) is good, the cusps (tips of teeth) of your lower jaw nestle securely into the fossa (valleys of teeth) of your upper jaw. That evenly spreads out the enormous biting forces you apply when eating.

If you have a class II malocclusion, however, then your upper teeth are not meeting the lower teeth correctly—they meet too far forward. This can cause cusp tip to hit against cusp tip—a situation that magnifies the forces applied to the cusps. When that happens, it can cause a fracture of the tooth. A fracture can be very painful and may take several visits to the dentist to fix. A fracture can even cause the tooth to die and need to be extracted. Class II malocclusion—also sometimes called bad bite—is one of the most common reasons for orthodontia.

7 REASONS TO STRAIGHTEN YOUR TEETH

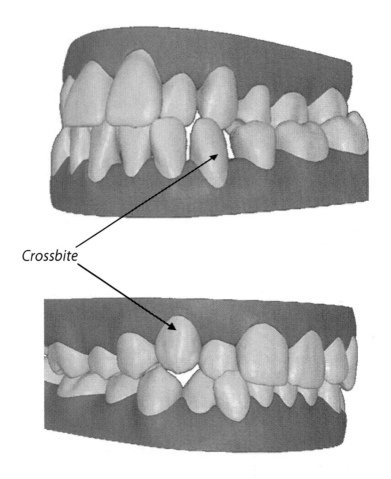

Crossbite

CROSSBITE

Your upper jaw is just a little bit larger than your lower jaw. It should be slightly longer and slightly wider. That is fortunate because it stops your teeth from banging into each other while you eat. Close your teeth now and look into a mirror. (I know you're not doing that now—but look later.) Normally, all of your upper teeth should be on the outside of your lower teeth.

If one or more of your upper teeth meet on the wrong side of your lower teeth, it's called a crossbite. Crossbites of the back teeth, called posterior crossbites, are more common. Crossbites of the front teeth are called anterior crossbites.

A posterior crossbite can interfere with normal chewing. It can often cause the person to unnaturally pull the jaw to the right or left in order to compensate for the bad bite. Such movements can stress the temporomandibular joint (the joint between your lower and upper jaws, often abbreviated as TMJ), as well as the tendons and muscles attached to the jaw. This can cause headaches, facial or jaw pain, and even limited movement of the joint. Posterior crossbite can also cause uneven wear on your tooth enamel, leading to an increased risk of cavities and fractured teeth.

An anterior crossbite can cause the affected teeth to become loose and can cause the gum to pull away from the root of the tooth.

7 REASONS TO STRAIGHTEN YOUR TEETH

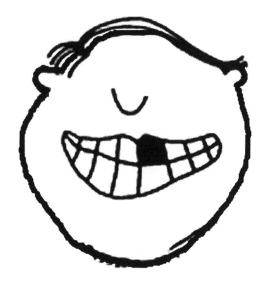

KNOCKED OUT TEETH

Accidents happen.

In fact, accidents happen more often than you think. Trauma is the number one cause of tooth loss in people under the age of 21.

In the event of an accident or other trauma, when a tooth is *avulsed* (knocked out of its socket), quick action and a plan may help ensure the tooth can be successfully re-implanted.

First, retrieve the avulsed tooth and hold it by the crown (not the root). If the tooth is dirty, gently rinse it off with water. Do not scrub it or remove any attached soft tissue. If possible, try to gently place the tooth back into its correct position. Do not use force. If you cannot replace the tooth, then put the tooth in a small container of milk (if milk is not available, then use water that contains a tiny pinch of table salt). Then see your dentist as quickly as possible.

Knocked-out teeth with the highest chances of being saved are those treated by a dentist and returned to their socket within an hour of being knocked out.

If your family dentist is unavailable, most hospital emergency rooms have a dentist on staff or available on call.

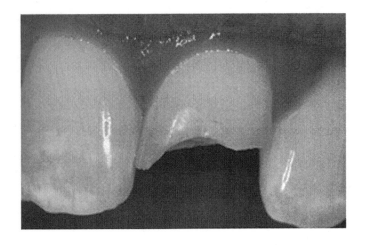

FRACTURED TEETH

Fractured (broken) teeth happen fairly often—there are a lot of ways to get hit in the mouth. Here's a list of the most common causes of fractured teeth:

- Ice hockey (2.3%)
- Motorcycle accidents (10.4%)
- Motor vehicle collisions (10.8%)
- Contact sports (15.9%)
- Altercations (17%)
- Unknown (17%)

Types of Fractured Teeth

Broken teeth fall into three classes:

- *Class I fractures* involve only the enamel; these injuries may show minor chipping with rough edges. These fractures are usually not painful.

- *Class II fractures* involve enamel and dentin; the tooth is usually painful if you touch it or expose it to air. The dentin may appear yellow. These fractures are more painful.

- *Class III fractures* involve the enamel, dentin, and pulp. These fractures will usually be very painful. You may see pinkish or reddish markings around the surrounding dentin or blood in the center of the tooth from the exposed pulp.

Any fractured tooth, even if it seems to be a Class I fracture, should be seen by a dentist as soon as possible. Repairing the tooth will help you keep it.

7 REASONS TO STRAIGHTEN YOUR TEETH

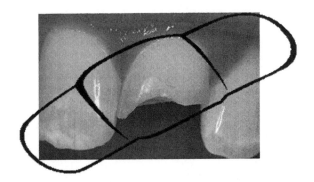

FIRST AID FOR FRACTURED TEETH

If you fracture a tooth, there's a reasonable chance a dentist can restore it if you can save the broken pieces. It's possible your dentist can cement all the pieces of tooth together and replace it in the socket. Whether or not you can find the pieces, follow these first aid steps for broken teeth:

- Rinse your mouth very nicely with warm water. If you have saved the tooth pieces, rinse those as well.

- Put gauze on the bleeding spot and leave it for 10 minutes or until the bleeding stops.

- Apply an ice pack to the lips and cheeks just over the broken tooth. This will lessen the pain and swelling.

- If you are unable to reach the dentist, cover the tooth temporarily with dental cement. This can be found in any drug store.

- Take over-the-counter pain relievers such as ibuprofen (Advil), aspirin, or acetaminophen (Tylenol).

7 REASONS TO STRAIGHTEN YOUR TEETH

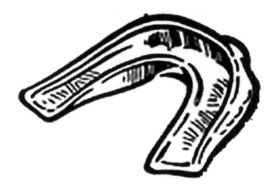

USE A MOUTH GUARD

Every day, baseballs, hockey pucks, lacrosse sticks, bicycles, automobiles and all sorts of other objects potentially threaten teeth. The primary cause of tooth loss of young people is trauma, but often that trauma could be avoided.

Most high school and college athletic coaches encourage the use of mouth guards during all contact sports. Think of mouth guards as safety belts for your teeth.

Your family dentist can fit you with a custom mouth guard, but effective premade mouth guards are easily available at drug stores and sporting good stores. The premade varieties cost only a few dollars. They may not last as long as the one your dentist makes for you, but they're still very effective. Replace the mouth guard if it becomes worn out or doesn't fit well anymore.

When it comes to protecting your teeth against accidental trauma the old saying, "An ounce of prevention is worth a pound of cure" is certainly true.

7 REASONS TO STRAIGHTEN YOUR TEETH

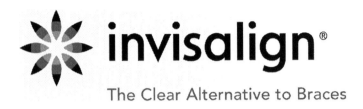

The Clear Alternative to Braces

7. Unexpected Benefits: The Invisalign Advantage

You've just read six good reasons to straighten your teeth. The seventh reason is unexpected benefits if you choose to straighten your teeth using *Invisalign*®: Things that will improve in your life even though they don't directly have anything to do with your teeth. We can't say for sure that any one of the unexpected benefits described here will happen to you—and it's possible you'll have an unexpected benefit that isn't discussed here. (If you do, please tell your dentist or orthodontist about it!)

7 REASONS TO STRAIGHTEN YOUR TEETH

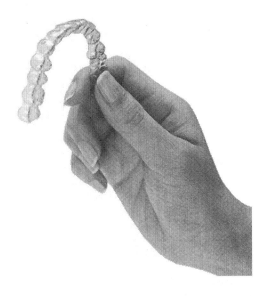

7. UNEXPECTED BENEFITS: THE INVISALIGN ADVANTAGE

WHAT IS *INVISALIGN*®?

The *Invisalign*® system is a way to straighten your teeth easily and nearly invisibly, without clumsy and unsightly metal braces. Here's how it works:

You wear a series of removable, clear, comfortable and virtually invisible aligners. Each aligner is individually manufactured for you using exact calculations. As you wear the aligners, they gently nudge your teeth into a better position. You wear the aligners 22 hours a day—all the time except when eating.

Each aligner is worn for about two weeks; as your teeth gradually move into position, you switch to a new aligner that will move them a bit more. As you move through your series of aligners, your teeth will progress from the position they are today to the final position. For most people, the whole process takes between six and eighteen months. Your smile and your dental health will be transformed effortlessly.

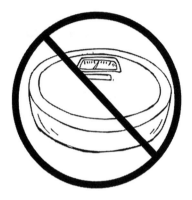

7. UNEXPECTED BENEFITS: THE INVISALIGN ADVANTAGE

WEIGHT LOSS WITHOUT DIETING

When you wear the *Invisalign*® aligners, you can talk and do all your normal activities without anyone noticing them. You do have to remove the aligners and store them in their case when you eat or drink anything except water or sugarless liquids. Before reinserting the aligners, you should brush your teeth—otherwise trapped sugar or food particles can increase the risk of cavities and gum disease. Because this is sometimes inconvenient, many *Invisalign*® patients find that they snack much less between meals. They look at the donut, think about having to brush after eating it, and decide to just skip it. Because between-meal eating tends to be heavy on fatty, sugary, high-calorie snacks, simply avoiding these foods automatically reduces the number of calories you take in every day. That means weight loss without really trying, to say nothing of better health from not eating nutritionally empty foods loaded with fat, sugar, and salt.

7 REASONS TO STRAIGHTEN YOUR TEETH

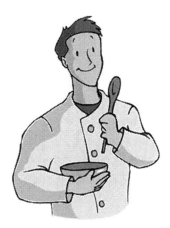

WEIGHT LOSS WITHOUT DIETING: FOLLOW CHEF TODD

I first realized this unexpected benefit from one of my patients. Chef Todd is well known and has a very popular restaurant. He began *Invisalign®* treatment because he was in the public eye. He wanted a nicer, warmer smile, but he didn't want to wear obvious metal braces on his teeth. He was also very busy with his restaurant and wanted a process that wasn't time-consuming or painful. *Invisalign®* was the obvious choice.

As a chef, Todd was exposed to great food all the time. Until he started wearing *Invisalign®*, however, he had no idea how often he snacked between meals. On his first day, he reached for an hôrs d'oeuvre and realized that to eat it, he would have to remove the aligners, brush, and reinsert them. That made him realize that he was constantly eating—he was always sneaking a cookie, a piece of bread, a slice of meat, a chunk of cheese, a handful of nuts, to say nothing of sampling what was cooking in his restaurant kitchen.

What the *Invisalign®* process taught him was to think before he snacked. It retrained his dietary habits. During his *Invisalign®* treatment, Chef Todd lost 40 pounds effortlessly. Even better, the aligners helped him break the snacking habit, and he has kept the weight off.

7 REASONS TO STRAIGHTEN YOUR TEETH

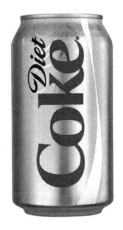

7. UNEXPECTED BENEFITS: THE INVISALIGN ADVANTAGE

GO SUGARLESS

Michael, one my teenaged patients, is a typical American boy. Unfortunately, that meant he was drinking two to three cans of regular *Coke* every day. A single can of *Coke* contains the equivalent of ten teaspoons of pure sugar, which means he was drinking two to three candy bars a day!

Michael was a typical teenage boy in another way, too—he was overweight. In the average teen diet, the single biggest source of added sugars and calories is sodas and fruit drinks. A 12-ounce can of *Coke* has 155 calories, which means Michael was taking in between 360 and 465 extra calories of sugar every day—enough for him to be gaining weight at the rate of nearly a pound a week. A study by the Harvard School of Public Health found that for each additional serving of soda or juice drink a child has each day, that child's chance of becoming overweight increases by 60 percent, which is exactly what was happening to Michael! Plus, all those sweetened drinks push out other, healthier foods from the diet and also lead to a much higher rate of cavities.

When Michael started wearing the *Invisalign*® aligners, he had a choice: He could remove the aligners and brush his teeth every time he had a *Coke* or some other sugary drink, or he could switch to the sugar-free versions. He switched.

The benefits of *Invisalign*® to Michael went beyond straight teeth. He not only lost weight, he got far fewer cavities, all from one simple change he had to make because of the aligners. As with Chef Todd, his weight loss was almost effortless.

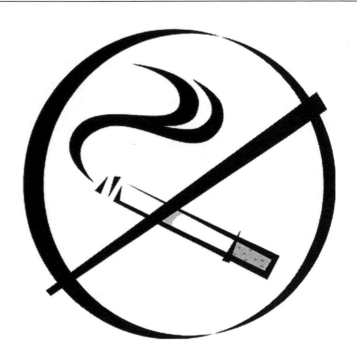

7. UNEXPECTED BENEFITS: THE INVISALIGN ADVANTAGE

NO SMOKING

You know that smoking is terrible for your lungs and heart, but did you know it's also terrible for your teeth? Tobacco products (including smokeless tobacco) stain your teeth, cause bad breath, and can cause oral cancer. Tobacco also harms your gums by constricting the tiny blood vessels that bring nutrients to your gums and teeth and by lowering your body's ability to fight off infection. Smokers get gum disease and lose teeth more often than nonsmokers. And because their bodies are less able to heal, treating gum disease in smokers is less effective.

Quitting smoking is extremely difficult. Very few smokers manage it the first time, and most take several tries before they can give up tobacco completely. But if you decide to straighten your teeth with *Invisalign®*, you'll have a strong incentive to give up smoking. After all, what's the point of having straight teeth if they still have horrible brown cigarette stains? And just as tobacco smoke stains your teeth, it may also stain the aligners. That takes away one of the best features about *Invisalign®*—invisibility. Smoking can also seriously affect your progress with *Invisalign®*. The poor circulation in your gums and surrounding tissue caused by smoking makes your teeth less responsive to the treatment.

When patients ask me if they can wear their *Invisalign®* aligners while smoking, I simply tell them that they shouldn't smoke, and this would be a fine time to quit!

7 REASONS TO STRAIGHTEN YOUR TEETH

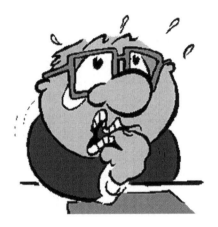

7. UNEXPECTED BENEFITS: THE INVISALIGN ADVANTAGE

NO MORE NAIL-BITING

An unexpected benefit of *Invisalign®* that really surprised me is that it helps stop nail-biting. Janice, one of my patients, was 39 and had been biting her nails for as long as she could remember. The habit was unsightly and distressing to her, and it was driving her husband crazy. She would bite her nails even when they were just having a conversation together. Janice would go for expensive manicures and promise herself that she wouldn't bite her nails afterward. Of course, the habit would kick in and she would wreck her nice nails all over again.

Shortly after she started wearing her first set of *Invisalign®* aligners, she unconsciously began biting her nails. She immediately realized that she couldn't chomp down on her nails while the aligners were in place. At first, she found this very disturbing—she even thought of removing the aligners for a few minutes so she could give in to her habit. She resisted, though, and was able to keep resisting as time went by.

Janice felt the aligners not only physically prevented her from biting her nails, they made her more aware of how unconscious the habit was. As with any bad habit, becoming aware of the problem is the first step toward breaking it. In this case, Janet was completely cured of her nail-biting. Even after she had completed the treatment, she never went back to chewing her nails.

7 REASONS TO STRAIGHTEN YOUR TEETH

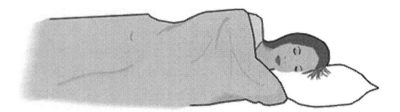

SLEEP BETTER

Grinding or clenching your teeth while you sleep—what dentists call *bruxism*—is a surprisingly common problem. Somewhere between 5 and 20 percent of all adults do it. Stress can make bruxism worse, but we don't really know what makes people grind and clench their teeth in their sleep.

Bruxism puts a lot of pressure on the muscles, tendons, and other structures around your jaw. This can cause painful temporomandibular joint problems (TMJ). It can also wear down your teeth and might even be noisy enough to wake someone else in the bedroom. If your teeth are maloccluded, bruxism is an even bigger problem, causing much more wear on the teeth. Tooth grinding can also lead to disrupted sleep, causing daytime tiredness and all the other problems associated with sleep disorders.

One common treatment for tooth grinding is a night guard, also called a mouth guard or splint. There are several different kinds of night guards, but the general idea for all of them is to create a barrier or cushion between the top and bottom teeth.

Invisalign® aligners are worn at night, which means they act as a night guard, keeping the upper and lower teeth apart. This unexpected benefit has helped many patients finally realize that their frequent jaw pain, earaches, and headaches are actually caused by nighttime tooth grinding. Once they've completed the *Invisalign*® treatment, they use *Invisalign Vivera*® retainers or night guards to control their bruxism.

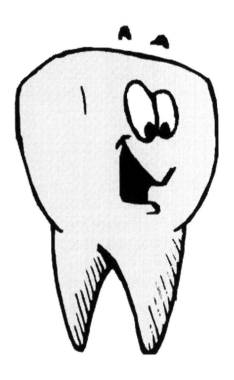

TOOTH JUNKIES

Many of my *Invisalign®* patients become what I call "tooth junkies." I mean that in a positive way, of course. They see their slow and steady progress as their teeth straighten. And as their teeth straighten, they notice that flossing become easier—and they then floss more. They notice that the redness in their gums begins to disappear and that their gums don't bleed as much when they brush— and they then brush more. They realize that their teeth aren't as white as they could be—and they get their teeth whitened.

What it all really comes down to is that they respect their teeth more. They feel better about themselves and they smile much more. They tell other people about their experience. They become ambassadors for better tooth care.

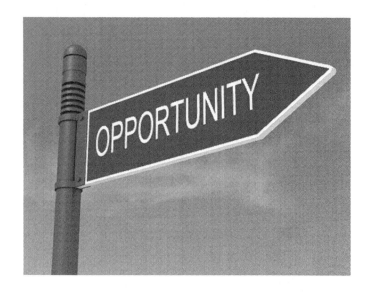

7. UNEXPECTED BENEFITS: THE INVISALIGN ADVANTAGE

PARTICIPATE IN YOUR OWN HEALTH CARE

Today, it's becoming increasingly important for people to participate in their own health care. Not only does this save money and trips to the doctor, but in the long run, those who take part in their own health care live longer, healthier lives. Eating right, exercising, good safety habits (such as wearing your seat belt) are all important ways that folks can take responsibility for their own health.

With *Invisalign®* therapy, the patient takes on most of the responsibility for his or her own treatment. It's up to the patient to wear the aligners as prescribed and to do the dental care that's necessary to make the treatment successful. By actively participating in their orthodontic treatment, patients realize how important it is to participate in other aspects of their overall health care as well. Many of my patients start taking better care of themselves in general. They tell me they stick to their medications better, because taking the pills becomes part of the regular health care regimen they have to do every day. They also follow up more on their health by keeping their doctor appointments and scheduling long-overdue preventive care such as physicals, colonoscopies and mammograms. Because of *Invisalign®*, they gain far more than just straight teeth!

7 REASONS TO STRAIGHTEN YOUR TEETH

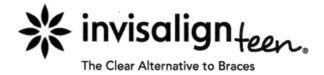

The Clear Alternative to Braces

MATURITY

Younger kids love regular braces, made with stainless steel brackets and wires. They like the colored rubber bands that hold the braces in place. The braces let them express their individualism and personality.

What kids like best about braces, however, is that they perceive them as a rite of passage. By wearing braces, they're moving from being little kids to big kids. They understand that they're now old enough to take on the responsibility of extra brushing and flossing that wearing braces require. Being seen as mature enough to take on that task is important to kids (although parents still have to check that proper dental care is really happening every day).

Teenagers, on the other hand, are frequently embarrassed by metal braces. They're moving into adulthood and are concerned (sometimes overly concerned) about their looks.

Everyone wants straight teeth. Kids want braces. Teens want *Invisalign*®. There is a specialized *Invisalign*® product for teenagers, appropriately called, *Invisalign Teen*®.

Teenagers, almost invariably, will choose *Invisalign Teen*® over braces for their orthodontic treatment. However, parents frequently want their adolescent to have traditional metal braces, thinking that their teen won't reliably cooperate with the *Invisalign*® program. They worry that their child won't wear the aligners long enough each day and would rather he or she had metal braces that can't be removed.

These worries are usually needless—my teenaged patients have usually been very responsible about wearing their aligners. In fact, *Invisalign Teen*® is an opportunity for teenagers to demonstrate maturity and prove to their parents that they're reliable. *Invisalign Teen*® is also an opportunity for teens to learn to actively participate in their own health care.

Invisalign Teen® is not only the clear way to give teens straight teeth; it is a window into adulthood.

SMILE!

Are you still wondering if you should straighten your teeth? Look at yourself in the mirror. Do you see crowded, crooked, or badly spaced teeth? If so, your smile isn't all it could be—and that means you aren't all you could be.

Teeth that aren't straight can cause serious dental problems. In fact, you may already have gum disease that's caused by the way your crooked teeth keep you from cleaning them effectively. We know that gum disease is directly related to other very serious health problems, including heart disease, stroke, and premature and low birth weight babies. A nice smile is good, but good health is even better.

Your sense of yourself as a worthwhile person can also be affected by your crooked teeth. When you don't feel good about your teeth, you don't feel good about yourself. Being self-conscious about your appearance can lead to feelings of low self-esteem. Crooked, crowded teeth may also make a poor first impression when you meet someone new, say for a job interview. By straightening your teeth, you strengthen your self-esteem and confidence.

Other good reasons for straightening your teeth include protecting them against accidental damage and cutting back on bad breath. You might even experience some unexpected benefits, such as weight loss, quitting smoking, and breaking other bad oral habits.

The reasons for straightening your teeth are compelling. Waiting only worsens your existing dental problems. Why delay? Your beautiful new smile is waiting for you.

ADDITIONAL RESOURCES

For more information, visit these websites:

www.braces.org

www.ada.org

www.cardodontics.com

www.Invisalign.com

www.Invisalignteen.com

www.brushyourteethbook.com

Dr. David Ostreicher's other book, *Brush Your Teeth! and other simple ways to stay young and healthy*, is available at amazon.com

ACKNOWLEDGEMENTS

I wish to thank my wife, Brenda, for her keen eye in proof reading this manuscript, and my daughters, Brie and Skye for their help with the artwork.

Made in the USA
Charleston, SC
21 July 2016